FIBROMYALGIA

The Ultimate Guide to Fibromyalgia and Chronic Fatigue, Including Fibromyalgia Symptoms, Medication, and How to Get Relief!

Table of Contents

Introduction

Thank you for taking the time to read this book: Fibromyalgia - The Ultimate Guide to Fibromyalgia and Chronic Fatigue, Including Fibromyalgia Symptoms, Medication and How to Get Relief!

Recent clinical surveys reveal that Fibromyalgia affects about 5% of the global population, which is approximately 350 million people. About 85% of Fibromyalgia patients are adult women, with the rest of the 15% being men and children.

Those who suffer from Fibromyalgia experience a wide range of symptoms, which include chronic pain, intensified receptivity to pain, stiffness of joints, and an inability to sleep. Even though not every patient manifests the same symptoms, these symptoms are considered to be the most common.

The specific cause of Fibromyalgia is still not fully known. However, there are many various theories about it. Some theories suggest that certain environmental factors could trigger the acquisition of Fibromyalgia.

There are theories that suggest that certain genes could elevate the risk of a person experiencing this medical condition. These genes are related to other medical disorders and syndromes including depression.

Even though medical experts are still not certain of the causes of Fibromyalgia, the good thing is there are proven and effective treatment methodologies that could make a significant difference to the life of the patient. Equipped with the right information, those who are suffering from Fibromyalgia can still pursue a healthy and satisfying life without the limitations imposed by this medical condition.

At the completion of this book you will have a good understanding of fibromyalgia, how it's diagnosed, treated, managed, and improved.

Once again, thanks for picking up this book. I hope you find it to be helpful!

Chapter 1:
Fibromyalgia: Common Symptoms and Possible Causes

Fibromyalgia is a medical disorder, which is characterized by pain in the muscles and joints, stress, lethargy, insomnia, and depression. According to recent studies, fibromyalgia could elevate the body's receptivity to pain because the disorder changes the brain's interpretation of pain.

Bear in mind that fibromyalgia is a syndrome which is characterized by a group of symptoms. When one or two symptoms are present in a person, it can be a sign of the presence of a particular disease or disorder. Below are the common symptoms in the case of fibromyalgia syndrome:

Lethargy

People with fibromyalgia often wake up feeling tired despite getting enough sleep at night. Sleep could be disturbed by pain, and most fibromyalgia patients are also suffering from sleep disorders, which include restless legs syndrome and sleep apnea. Fatigue could be mild to severe, and may leave patients feeling exhausted all day. There are times that patients may feel tired even if they have not done any work all day. Sudden fatigue is also evident, which leaves you unable to perform your tasks.

General Pain

The pain caused by fibromyalgia is often distinguished by a long-lasting dull pain, which may last for 2 to 3 months. General pain refers to the widespread body ache above and below your waist, and on both sides of the body, but it can be worse in a specific body area. It is likely that pain is ever-present, even though it is likely to worsen or ease off at various times. The type of pain that patients experience may also differ. Some experience stabbing, sharp pains, while other feel a burning sensation.

Headache

Any patient who often experience stiffness and pain in their neck and shoulders could also experience headaches. The headaches could be mild, but some patients also report experiencing migraines.

Fibro Fog

Fibromyalgia is also related to fibro fog, which affects the person's ability to focus, pay attention and accomplish mental tasks with ease. Therefore, learning and thinking could be affected, and speech could also be a bit confused and slow.

Stiffness

Fibromyalgia can make patients feel that they are very stiff, specifically if they have been lying or sitting in the same position for an extended period of time. Stiffness could be quite extreme upon waking, and moving to ease the stiffness may cause muscular spasms.

Hyperalgesia

Hyperalgesia, or high sensitivity, is usually present in patients suffering from fibromyalgia. This symptom could lead to sustaining pain when you are touched or you have bruised your arm, when in normal circumstances you should not feeling pain. This symptom is also known as Allodynia.

Sleep Problems

Fibromyalgia could also affect the patient's sleeping patterns. The condition could prevent the patient from falling into a restful sleep and this leaves patients tired.

Irritable Bowel Syndrome (IBS)

IBS may cause digestion problems such as constipation, diarrhea, and bloating. Many fibromyalgia patients also have a bloated tummy.

Depression

Many patients who are suffering from fibromyalgia also experience depression, and this is primarily because the symptoms of this disorder can be difficult to deal with. Some research also suggests that having a limited level of certain hormones could also make patients more prone to depression.

Other Symptoms

Additional symptoms that could be experienced by fibromyalgia patients may include painful periods, dizziness, paresthesia (numbness in the hands), anxiety, and an inability to control your body temperature.

Why Women Are More Prone to Fibromyalgia

It is interesting to note that women are more prone to suffer from fibromyalgia compared to men. Based on the recent statistics from the National Institutes of Health, around 85% of patients with this disorder are women.

Researchers suggest that this could have something to do with the hormones of women, differences in the immune system as well as the genes. But until now, there is no established fact yet as to why women are at high vulnerability of experiencing this disorder.

Fibromyalgia Causes

Despite of the many medical research advancements, scientists are still not certain about the causes of fibromyalgia. But doctors believe that the disorder may likely relative to various factors such as infections, genetics, and physical or emotional trauma.

Infection

Many people who experience fibromyalgia also acquire forms of viral and bacterial infection, which could be worsened by the syndrome. Patients with active infections are at a high risk of acquiring more infections, particularly bacterial infections that could lead to further health problems. Some fibromyalgia patients are more vulnerable to any type of infection because the condition can affect the immune system. Hence, it is important for the doctor to identify the various factors to ascertain if the infection is a consequence, an aggravator, or a main cause of the disorder.

Genetics

It is important to take note that fibromyalgia is not directly transmitted from parents to their offspring. However, the syndrome sometimes appears to occur in clusters within families. The risk of getting fibromyalgia is higher in the immediate relatives of people with the disorder than the families without a history of the disease.

DNA plays a vital role in the nervous system's response to pain. There are genes that are linked with depression and anxiety, which could be the reason why certain medications for depression occasionally help in easing out particular fibromyalgia symptoms.

Trauma

Physical injury could lead to post-traumatic fibromyalgia. Medical specialists in fibromyalgia report that many of their patients experienced symptoms after a major physical injury. About 60% of fibromyalgia cases are caused by whiplash injury.

Pain Caused by Fibromyalgia

The pain that is often related to fibromyalgia is characterized as widespread, which means you can feel pain above and below the waist as well as on both sides of your body.

Some patients also report pain in specific areas of the body, which they could feel the pain even if they take pain relievers. Joints and muscles might feel like they have been overworked or have been pulled, even though there is no laborious work occurring. There are even cases of muscular twitching. In some instances, the patient may feel a burning sensation with a sharp stabbing ache. Some fibromyalgia patients may also feel pain surrounding the joints in their back, hips, neck, and shoulders. This kind of pain is often the main cause of inability to sleep and exercise.

Fibromyalgia pain is regarded as chronic because the pain may last much longer than it is commonly expected. The pain could be unending, and the lasting back pain, neck pain, joint pain, and headache could affect normal sleeping patterns. Lack of sleep could result in elevated pain, lethargy, and stiffness. Although the patient may want to perform exercise or do daily tasks, it might be impossible because of the pain in the joints, knees, legs, and hips. Fibromyalgia pain can leave sufferers incapacitated, so their ability to work and have fun is quite limited.

The chronic pain could lead to irritation. Hence, the patient may find it a challenge to deal with other people. Since fibromyalgia primarily affects women, it is often difficult for them to take care of their children while working. Without proper diagnosis, the patient fails to find the right treatment, the symptoms may lead to lethargy, social isolation, depression, irritability, and anxiety.

Chapter 2:
How to Get Diagnosis for Fibromyalgia

You may have already consulted a doctor who has identified your condition as fibromyalgia. But this condition is a tricky one to diagnose. Hence, it is best for patients and their loved ones to review the proper diagnosis, as there are often cases of suspected fibromyalgia that turn out to be other medical conditions such as Chronic Fatigue Syndrome, which you will later learn about later in this chapter.

Because of multi-faceted treatment methods that include lifestyle strategies and medications, the prognosis for individuals suspected to have fibromyalgia is now better. However, the doctor should first make a precise fibromyalgia diagnosis.

Fibromyalgia is often misunderstood and as such, patients with similar symptoms suffer misdiagnosis. In spite of all the latest research results and information concerning fibromyalgia, doctors still find it challenging to diagnose this common physical disorder. Hence, some patients are getting diagnosed for the wrong medical condition.

Why Is It Difficult to Diagnose Fibromyalgia?

Fibromyalgia is composed of symptoms that are also present in many other medical conditions. Doctors should rule out the other conditions before finally diagnosing fibromyalgia. There is no simple medical examination to diagnose fibromyalgia. Many patients visit several doctors without receiving proper diagnosis for the symptoms that they experience. Some even suspect that their symptoms are simply imagined.

Previously, many fibromyalgia patients were misdiagnosed as having systemic exertion intolerance disease, chronic myofascial pain, lupus or rheumatoid, inflammatory arthritis, or even mere depression. Of course, there are similar symptoms, but fibromyalgia is a different condition. This is a distinct condition that requires precise diagnosis and proper treatment.

Types of Medical Exams Used for Fibromyalgia Diagnosis

Many lab tests are useful for fibromyalgia diagnosis. One test that is often used by doctors is the FM/a. This is a blood test that helps in identifying markers released by the blood cells in the immune system of people with fibromyalgia. One research shows that this test could help in identifying fibromyalgia from other conditions, which could have similar symptoms such as lupus or rheumatoid arthritis.

A doctor will often make a diagnosis after performing a physical exam. He or she will also discuss the symptoms with you, because a large percentage of the diagnosis is based on what you feel. For example, although the doctor may observe tender areas during the physical exam, the patient must also describe the doctor about the pain that they feel.

In order to make certain that the patient doesn't have a more severe medical case, the doctor will also perform more laboratory exams. These exams could probably be performed during a single visit to a laboratory.

Your doctor may require you to take a complete blood count (CBC), which measures the platelets, white cells, red cells, and hemoglobin. This could also find other common blood disorders such as anemia, which can also cause lethargy.

There are also cases that the doctor may require additional tests such as liver and kidney tests to check blood chemistries. It is also important to know the levels of calcium, cholesterol and other types of fats in your bloodstream. Furthermore, your doctor may also perform thyroid tests to check if your thyroid is underactive or overactive.

Test for Inflammatory Arthritis

A doctor who is diagnosing fibromyalgia often tests the sedimentation rate of the red blood cells. This specific test provides a rough index of inflammation in the body. In inflammatory arthritis, this test is not normal. It could also be abnormal with some types of infection. This is usually normal in cases of fibromyalgia and osteoarthritis.

The patient may also be required to be tested for anti-CCP antibodies and rheumatoid factor. These blood tests together could help in the diagnosis of about 79% of patients with inflammatory arthritis.

The doctor may also require test for anti-nuclear antibodies or ANA. Similar to the rheumatoid factor, the ANA is strange antibody in the blood, which is usually found in people with systemic lupus. The latter condition is very common in younger women and may also cause fatigue and pain. This condition may also result to problems in the internal organs such as brain problems, heart problems, and kidney disease.

X-Ray and Fibromyalgia

More often than not, the x-ray scans of areas that are painful will show no sign of abnormality for people with fibromyalgia. If the patient is suffering from another condition such as arthritis, then there could be some abnormalities on the X-rays showing the type of arthritis that the patient has. Bear in mind that any changes in the X-ray scans are not caused by fibromyalgia.

Which Test Could Rule Out Severe Medical Problems?

It is important that the patient openly talks about the condition with the doctor to understand the general results of the diagnosis. You can ask your doctor to explain the results of the physical exam, the x-rays, and the lab tests. Through this, you can understand fibromyalgia even better. Don't hesitate to ask questions about this medical condition, including the symptoms and the types of treatments you can undergo.

Fibromyalgia Diagnostic Guidelines

When other severe medical conditions have been ruled out by the initial exams, the doctor will consider if your conditions are within the criteria for fibromyalgia:

- Widespread pain (above and below the waist, and in both sides of the body)

- Pain has been experienced for at least three months

- Other possible diseases that may cause the pain have been ruled out

Other Medical Problems That Will Be Assessed in Fibromyalgia Diagnosis

In order to be thorough when it comes to diagnosing fibromyalgia, the doctor will perform the following:

- Examine for widespread pain

- Assess body trigger points

- Ask questions about fatigue

- Ask questions about sleep problems

- Assess your stress level

- Examine for depression

Once your condition has been confirmed to be fibromyalgia, your doctor will talk about the multi-faceted treatment options. The treatment program may involve prescription drugs, exercises, stress relief strategies, sleep techniques, and even alternative medicines. Sticking to the program will help the patient to alleviate the symptoms of fibromyalgia.

Fibromyalgia and Chronic Fatigue Syndrome (CFS)

Chronic Fatigue Syndrome (CFS) is commonly related to fibromyalgia, because the symptoms are usually the same. Like fibromyalgia, patients with CFS also feel tiredness on a level which they find it hard to perform their everyday activities. Even though the cause of CFS is still not known and could be difficult to diagnose, many of the symptoms could be treated.

Causes of CFS

Similar to fibromyalgia, the causes of CFS are also not certain. In some instances, patients experience CFS after suffering physical or emotional trauma or after prolonged exposure to toxins. The main cause of CFS is still unknown.

Medical specialists suggest the possible causes of CFS as being: genetics, hormonal imbalance, and weakened immune system. However, it is crucial to take note that there is not enough established fact to declare that these factors cause CFS.

Symptoms of CFS

CFS Symptoms usually manifest immediately. But for some people, they slowly develop over a span of weeks. The symptoms may vary from day to day, and there is the tendency that the CFS symptoms may suddenly disappear (remission) and then will start to occur again (relapse).

There are several types of CFS symptoms, but there are core sets, which may appear on people suffering from this syndrome. The following are the main symptoms of CFS.

Physical and Mental Fatigue

Patients with CFS experience constant tiredness or it could be recurring. This cannot be relieved by resting, and it can affect their everyday activities.

Sudden Weakness After A Strenuous Activity

This CFS symptom refers to being very weak or ill after performing laborious tasks such as swimming, running, or exercising. The weakness is usually sudden, and it may take several days for the patient to restore their strength.

Pain

The pain that is related to CFS might be isolated or widespread. In some instances, the pain may only be felt in one area, and then transfer to another. The patient could suffer from headaches, joint pain, or muscle pain. In some cases, the pain could be so severe that the patient may experience sleep problems as a result.

Other Symptoms

CFS patients could also experience feeling disoriented, light sensitivity, confusion, lack of focus, and short-term memory problems. In some instances, the patients can also experience sudden changes in their weight, irritable bowel syndrome (IBS), urinating, nausea, shortness of breath when doing strenuous activities, lightheadedness, and dizziness.

What Are the Differences Between CFS and Fibromyalgia?

More often than not, doctors treat fibromyalgia and CFS separately, while many think that they are just the same disorder, or a variety of fibromyalgia. According to research, approximately 65% of patients diagnosed with fibromyalgia also have CFS.

CFS and fibromyalgia are both known to show main symptoms including impaired coordination, dizziness, cognitive impairment, IBS, chronic headache, lack of sleep, fatigue, and pain.

One primary difference when it comes to diagnosis is which among the symptoms are manifesting the most and the worst - pain or lethargy. The diagnosis could even be affected by the familiarity of the doctor to these diseases. However, researchers have also distinguished core differences. Many cases of CFS manifest after experiencing flu-like symptoms and can even be caused and aggravated by a viral infection.

Patients of CFS also show activation of a chronic immune system, which signifies that the body is combating the infection. This is not true in fibromyalgia. Moreover, the diagnostic factor for CFS includes a low-grade fever and sore throat. These symptoms are not considered when diagnosing fibromyalgia. Meanwhile, the onset of fibromyalgia is often traced to a physical or emotional trauma. The pain associated with fibromyalgia can get be eased out with a soothing massage, while CFS pain cannot be eased through this treatment.

Chapter 3:
Prescription Drugs for Fibromyalgia

The medication-based treatment for fibromyalgia is symptom-based, which means that the medication to take depends on the main set of symptoms experienced by the patient. There are medications used to treat symptoms such as antidepressants, sleeping pills, and pain. There are also medications used to help in easing the pain, while others can help in improving sleep and in boosting mood. It is crucial for you to work with your doctor so you can find the right medication for your fibromyalgia symptoms. This way, you can effectively manage your symptoms.

Fibromyalgia Initial Treatment

Antidepressants are the initial prescription drugs that doctors usually recommend for fibromyalgia patients. These drugs help in the relief of fatigue, pain, and sleep difficulties. Moreover, antidepressants could help in depression, which is often experienced by fibromyalgia patients. Classic antidepressants such as tricyclics have been prescribed by doctors for many years to treat fibromyalgia.

Tricyclic Antidepressants in the Treatment of Fibromyalgia

Tricyclic antidepressants such as nortiphtyline and amitriptyline are prescribed to increase the levels of neurotransmitters in the brain. These antidepressants increase the neorepinephrine and serotonin levels in the brain. Patients who experience chronic pain usually have decreased levels of these relaxing neurotransmitters. Tricyclics could calm painful muscles and elevate the effects of endorphins, which are the natural painkillers of the body. Although these prescription drugs are usually effective, there are side effects too like constipation, dry eyes, dry mouth, dizziness, and drowsiness.

Pain and Fatigue Relief Using Antidepressants

There are various types of antidepressants, which have been observed to help in the relief of pain, fatigue, and sleep problems among fibromyalgia patients. The highly noted antidepressants for fibromyalgia are venlafaxine, milnacipran, and duloxetine. Brand names for duloxetine (Cymbalta) and milnacipran (Savella) are particularly approved by the FDA to treat fibromyalgia. There are still limited studies on the effects of venlafaxine (Effexor) in its efficacy for fibromyalgia. Other medications that could also help in the relief of fibromyalgia symptoms are Paxil (pareotine), Prozac (fluoxetine), and Celexa (citalopram).

Various antidepressants have different effects on the body. Moreover, what works for one fibromyalgia patient may not work for another patient. Hence, you may need to try several types of antidepressants to find the best drug that could relieve the pain, sleep problems, and fatigue that are connected with the condition. Some doctors may even prescribe a combination of several antidepressants.

Prescription Drug to Help in the Relief of Fibromyalgia Pain

Various kinds of pain relievers are often recommended to soothe the pain emanating from trigger points or those coming from deep muscles caused by fibromyalgia. But the downside is, many of these painkillers usually don't work for all patients with fibromyalgia.

Over-the-counter drugs such as acetaminophen increase the threshold for pain, so the body will perceive less pain.

When taken alone, Non-Steroidal Anti-Inflammatory Drugs (NSAIDs) are not usually effective for the treatment of fibromyalgia symptoms. But when taken with other prescription drugs for fibromyalgia, NSAIDs such as Aleve (naproxen), ibuprofen (Advil), and aspirin (Motrin) can be effective.

Pain Reliever Side Effects of Pain Relievers for Fibromyalgia

You should take extra caution in taking NSAIDs, particularly aspirin, if you have stomach conditions. NSAIDs could result in stomach bleeding, stomach ulcers, vomiting, nausea or heartburn. There is also a higher risk for severe stomach bleeding for people who are more than 60 years old. It is not ideal to take NSAIDs for more than 2 weeks without consulting the doctor. These drugs have been observed to increase the risk of stroke and heart attack, particularly if taken in high dosages. Aspirin has been noted to trigger stomach ulcers. Be sure to consult your doctor about taking NSAIDs, if you have any type or intestinal or stomach bleeding in the past.

Meanwhile, acetaminophen has no known side effects. However, you should stay away from this medication if you have liver problems. Over-dosage could result in serious liver damage.

Muscle Relaxants for the Treatment of Fibromyalgia Pain

Muscle relaxants such as cyclobenzaprine have been proven to be effective for the treatment of fibromyalgia. This is usually recommended by doctors to help in soothing muscle tension and help in improving sleep problems. Muscle relaxants can also affect the levels of chemicals to relax muscles.

Muscle relaxants also have their own side effects, which include change in urine color, unsteadiness, clumsiness, blurry vision, drowsiness, dizziness, and dry mouth. These prescription drugs may also increase the likelihood of seizures. There are also cases of older adults experiencing hallucinations and confusion when taking them.

Anticonvulsants for Fibromyalgia Pain

Anticonvulsants, also known as anti-seizure drugs, are also used for the treatment of fibromyalgia. These drugs, such as Lyrica (pregabalin) were originally used for the treatment of seizures. When it comes to fibromyalgia, pregabalin affects the brain chemicals, which send pain receptors throughout the nervous system. This could reduce fatigue and pain and helps in improving sleep.

Neurontin (gabapentin) is another antioseizure drug, which has been proven to ease symptoms associated with fibromyalgia.

Other Medications Used for Fibromyalgia

Pain killers like Ultram (tramadol) are also used in the treatment of fibromyalgia. This narcotic-like prescription drug triggers in the brain to influence the perception of pain. This is not, however, addictive like narcotics.

Furthermore, doctors also prescribe benzodiazepines like Xanax (alprazolam), Klonopin (clonazepam), Valium (diazepam) and Ativan (lorazepam) to ease out painful muscles, help the patient to fall asleep, and to treat restless legs syndrome, which is a distinct feeling in the legs that encourages the person to constantly move them. However, taking benziodiazepines should be controlled as they can be addictive. Over-dosage increases the risk of severe side effects.

Strong narcotic drugs like Vicodin (acetaminophen/hydrocodone), Percocet (acetaminophen/oxycodone), OxyContin (oxycodone), and Lortab (hydrocodone) are also prescribed if other medications and alternative treatments have been tried with no success. But they should be strictly controlled, as they are habit forming and can bring serious side effects.

Chapter 4:
Recommended Exercises
for Fibromyalgia

Most people who are first diagnosed with fibromyalgia are convinced that they should stay in bed. However, doctors will usually recommend some form of exercise.

Some patients who experience extreme pain and lethargy may have to exercise while still in bed. Slowly, they can work up to walk a few meters and back to bed, then to more fitted exercise such as treadmills. Exercise is crucial in managing the symptoms of fibromyalgia.

In this chapter, you will learn a step-by-step plan for starting your own exercise program to treat fibromyalgia.

Step 1: Understand that Exercise is Vital in the Treatment of Fibromyalgia

Doctors agree that exercise is a crucial aspect of an effective fibromyalgia treatment plan, because it encompasses the treatment of major fibromyalgia symptoms such as sleep problems, fatigue, and pain.

Exercise could help in increasing the body's strength, reduce stress, improve balance and sustain bone density. Regular exercise could also help in controlling weight, which is crucial to alleviate fibromyalgia pain.

If you have fibromyalgia; exercising and doing strenuous tasks may be last on your list of priorities, but you need to keep in mind that it could really help.

Step 2: Take It Slow

Regardless if you have been running triathlons or you have never moved a muscle before, the secret is to begin with small steps and slowly increase the level of your activity. Many fibromyalgia patients will need to start very slowly.

You should think of exercise like a form of medication, which starts out with a low dosage and increase gradually. For instance, you could begin walking just three minutes every day for one week, and then add another minute every week until you hit 20 to 30 minutes. It could take a while to reach this point, but this is fine.

For those who are not familiar with exercising, you should not call it exercise. Instead, change your mindset and call it being active, by doing things such as walking in the park, or lifting weights. It might be a challenge to move your body at first, but as you go on, you will notice that exercising will become easier.

Based on a 2010 study, regular every day activities like gardening, doing house chores, and taking the stairs can help in managing the pain and enhance every day body functions of fibromyalgia patients. This study is proof that every bit of activity can help in managing pain caused by fibromyalgia.

Step 3: Observe Your Body

If you were physically active before you were diagnosed with fibromyalgia, you might need to get to know another approach to exercising. Some people try to do too much too soon, and then they are often disappointed once their symptoms worsen.

Those who were athletic before should know how to observe their body and get used to taking smaller steps compared to before. As time passes by, the patient will learn the level of exercise that is right for them.

Step 4: Move Every Day

It is crucial to perform exercises and move your body every day in order to get the most benefit. For most patients, the best option is to use exercise equipment or walk, because these are the activities that can easily be performed.

Warm pool exercise is also an ideal way to start being active. This method has a calming effect on the joints and muscles and could help in managing the pain. But even if you begin in a pool, it is still recommended to eventually shift to a dry-ground workout. In addition, some people don't have access to a warm pool all throughout the year, so this could be difficult to sustain.

Among the activities that could help in easing the symptoms of fibromyalgia are low-impact exercise classes, strength training, yoga, running, and cycling.

The essential key here is to look for a type of exercise that you truly enjoy. You can visit your friends, walk your pet, and take a walk in the park. It could also be helpful if you have a friend or a family member to accompany you during your exercise routines.

Step 5: Change Your Exercise Routine

Regardless of whether you are participating in an exercise class or you are walking, the following exercise tips could help you manage pain or injury:

- Choose to exercise at the time of the day that you are feeling best. For many fibromyalgia patients, the ideal time is between 9 am to 4 pm. However, your ideal time may vary.

- Be sure to do some stretching, because this could reduce the pain after exercise and could warm up joints and muscles. It is possible to stretch while you are sitting, standing, or lying down. Some patients can even stretch while taking a shower or having a warm bath.

- Do some small steps first. When you are walking, you may want to avoid first swinging your arms or taking large strides. Also walk on even, flat surface to prevent your risk of stumbling.

- Transition into strength training. For strength routines, you can choose to perform elastic band exercises rather than weights and begin with a single set of repetitions.

- Take a pace. In performing strengthening or stretching exercises, you should alternate sides regularly and don't forget to take enough rest in between reps.

- Take enough rest. Again, be sure to feel and observe your body. If you need to take a rest, then take a rest. Remember, this is not a competition but a vital aspect of a fibromyalgia treatment plan.

- Reward yourself. Once you are done exercising, you can pamper yourself. Watch your favorite TV show or take a hot bath.

Step 6: Learn Patience

Even though exercise could improve fibromyalgia symptoms, the effects are not always immediate. Exercise is usually the best long-term treatment for fatigue and pain caused by fibromyalgia. However, it may take up to several months before you can observe an improvement in the symptoms.

You should work slowly and be patient. It may seem strenuous to reach your goals. However, as you slowly improve your movements, you will feel better and you will notice changes in the symptoms. Bear in mind that exercise is a vital part of your journey towards freedom from fibromyalgia pain.

Exercise versus Daily Activities

Daily activities and exercises are crucial components of a holistic treatment plan for fibromyalgia. Even though they have similarities, each one refers to particular forms of physical activity across a broad spectrum.

Physical activities refer to physical actions that you perform as a component of your daily life. This is usually unplanned and happens as a result of raising kids, travelling, or working - just living your life. Even though daily activities could be more laborious compared to other forms of activities, you can perform them without having your symptoms worsen. And similar to patterned exercise, these have been proven to enhance fatigue and pain.

On the other hand, exercise involves physical actions, which employs repetitive movements of large muscle groups to enhance the bodies fitness. Usually, exercise is patterned by the type of activity, intensity, and amount of time. Strength training, aerobic exercise, and flexibility training are vital elements of a holistic fitness routine.

More often than not, you may engage in both daily activities and exercise over the duration of your life depending on your schedule and your goals. The results are cumulative. To put this simply, it all just adds up. Small portions of activities throughout the day are far superior to idle living. There is a higher chance of feeling better over time through living an active lifestyle, and you will have more energy to be with your family, improve yourself, or focus at work as a result.

Selecting the Ideal Activities for Fibromyalgia

In general, there is no ideal activity for fibromyalgia. However, you should take note that performing activities, no matter how less intense, is way better than zero activities. Select activities that you can also enjoy or at least you find tolerable as well as locations that are close to your home or at work. This allows you to start easily and of course to stick with the routine.

In selecting activities, you should be cautious of your physical restrictions and make necessary changes to suit your needs. There are different ways that you can do this, which include minimizing the intensity of your movement. For instance, if a workout routine requires you to run for a few meters, you can instead substitute running with walking. If a treadmill is too strenuous on your muscles and joints, you can instead try a warm pool or stationary bike. Minor changes such as these could make activities more convenient so you can easily perform them and take advantage of the exercises.

If you want to consider adding a structured exercise to your routine, begin with aerobic activities such as bicycling, running, swimming, and walking. These activities will increase your breathing and heart rate, including your body temperature, so you will sweat. These are normal responses to exercise. Usually, aerobic activities lead to the best rewards for your fibromyalgia symptoms. You can later on add strength and flexibility training after your body has already adapted to the general intensity of your activities.

Be More Physically Active

There are no strict rules when it comes to becoming physically active. Numerous factors could affect where you start and how you could progress, like your energy levels at a specific time, your life schedule, the activities available for you, and many more.

There are two important factors to consider when integrating exercise into your daily activities: (1) Understanding how to properly exercise to avoid overexertion or injury and (2) Knowing how you can slowly progress so that your established habit becomes a long-term routine.

When you begin to intensify your activity, regardless if it is for the first time in your life or after you take a break from your usual routine, you should always remember to go slow and start low.

It is fine to push yourself a bit. Physical activity must be more intense compared to what your body is accustomed to so your fibromyalgia symptoms will improve. For example, you will notice that when you first begin walking, a single lap around a block may feel difficult. However, after several weeks of continuous walking, the same walk will not feel quite as hard.

When you reach this point, you have already adapted to the demands of completing a single lap and your body is now ready to level up the intensity. This will not happen after one day, but you will eventually achieve it, as long as you stay consistent. It is all up to you. You need to decide what to do and how much effort are you willing to exert. You can help yourself feel better by pursuing an active lifestyle.

Ten Things to Remember If You Are Exercising for Fibromyalgia

1. Slowly add lifestyle activity into your regular schedule. If you are trying to achieve too much too soon, you will be vulnerable to falling short of your goals, symptom flare-ups, and you could be injured.

2. It is not always easy to start an exercise program. It will take time to establish a routine, and feel comfortable with it.

3. During the first few days, you could feel tired and your body may feel sore after an increase in your physical activity levels. However, you should not give up. Take note that this is normal. Soreness based on activity will eventually fade away.

4. Once stimulated by physical activity. Your body will adapt, improve and grow.

5. If you're performing aerobic activities, you might be a bit winded or experience shortness of breath when you are exercising. Take note that this is normal. However, panting and hyperventilation is not normal and you should immediately seek medical attention.

6. If your fibromyalgia symptoms suddenly flare up, you should avoid strenuous activities for a while. But still,

you should continue being active. If you are experiencing a symptom flare, minimize your exercise time by at least 50 per cent.

7. Your goals should be achievable and small when you are just starting out. This may include being active for 10 minutes every day, participating in an aerobics class two times a week, or performing basic yoga.

8. Your long-term goals may be lofty, but starting slow is the key. Don't push too hard, too fast!

9. Always seek medical attention if you feel nausea, experience vomiting, hyperventilation, and other non-normal symptoms.

10. Don't stop exercising to manage your fibromyalgia symptoms.

Chapter 5:
Proper Nutrition for
Fibromyalgia Patients

Many fibromyalgia patients have reported experiencing symptoms after consuming certain foods, and even though many of the studies are still in their early stages, there is evidence that suggest that a simple diet can help patients in managing fibromyalgia symptoms, particularly fatigue and pain.

Managing fibromyalgia can pose a challenge, and the improvements are often incremental. Many conventional doctors choose prescription drugs like antidepressants and analgesics, which may lead to side effects.

A doctor who prefers nutritional wellness, is more likely to prescribe a biochemical treatment for fibromyalgia patients in order to identify the underlying causes that could be treated with safe nutritional therapies. It is an established fact that fibromyalgia is a complicated medical condition with no simple treatment. But if you look at a holistic body approach with natural supplements and a healthy lifestyle and diet, it is still possible to harness your body's natural healing abilities.

Here are the nutritional tips for fibromyalgia patients. Just make sure to consult your physician before you make any changes in your diet.

Avoid Additives

Food additives like monosodium glutamate (MSG) and aspartame, could act as excitoxin molecules that could trigger neurons increasing the body's receptivity to pain.

Fibro doctors agree that avoiding additives can help in decreasing fibromyalgia symptoms.

Increase Vitamin D Intake

Many of us don't get enough Vitamin D, which is important for fibromyalgia patients. Vitamin D deficiency can cause symptoms similar to those of fibromyalgia. Therefore, patients should be tested for Vitamin D deficiency before being diagnosed. Based on studies, this deficiency may lead to muscle and joint pain, and adding your Vitamin D intake can help. Physicians recommend taking Vitamin D supplements, especially during cold season. Foods that are naturally rich in Vitamin D are dairy products, tofu, whole grain cereals, fish oils, and mushrooms.

Minimize Caffeine Intake

Take note that fibromyalgia patients often experience sleep problems. Hence, some patients are enticed to load up coffee to obtain more energy to complete their tasks for the day. But this is not a great idea. Some people are drinking coffee so they can compensate for not getting sufficient sleep at night. If you are drinking coffee, particularly several hours before bed time, it could affect your sleep patterns. Rather than coffee, you could drink green tea, which is also a good source of antioxidants.

Add Fish Intake

Fatty fish like mackerel, sardines, herring, and salmon are naturally rich in Omega-3 fatty acids that are known to have anti-inflammatory properties and can help in avoiding cardiovascular disease. Increasing your consumption of these specific fish could help in minimizing pain brought by fibromyalgia. You should also increase intake of other foods that are rich in omega-3 fatty acids such as flax seed, oatmeal, cereal, and walnuts.

Munch on Vegetables

Some physicians suggest that oxidative stress could lead to enhanced fibromyalgia symptoms. Oxidative stress is a condition where the body is not generating enough antioxidants to combat free radicals. Vegetables are naturally rich in important antioxidants like Vitamin A, C, and E that fight free radicals.

Glutathione

Glutathione is the primary antioxidant released by the body to protect it from oxidative damage as well as to support the liver's detox process. Clinical studies reveal that patients with those with low levels of glutathione are more vulnerable to morning stiffness. You can get enough glutathione by taking supplements, but if you like all natural sources, you should consume more garlic, cruciferous vegetables, and eggs. These have high levels of sulfur, which is the main component of glutathione.

Chapter 6:
Stress Relief Strategies for Fibromyalgia Patients

Emotional stress can greatly influence your perception and receptivity of pain. That is why fibromyalgia patients are more vulnerable to stress compared to people who are not suffering from this condition.

Basically, stress weakens your body. A weak body is more vulnerable to the symptoms of fibromyalgia like depression, fatigue, and chronic pain. Doctors believe that if you try to eliminate specific stressful triggers from your life, it is possible for the body to experience reduced symptoms of fibromyalgia.

However, taking a break from every day stress is not as easy as it may seem. More often than not, fibromyalgia patients are overloaded with family and work obligations. Regardless of the situation, most people with fibromyalgia are not taking care of themselves first.

Specific changes in everyday living like taking time to relax and prioritizing health are crucial aspect of managing fibromyalgia.

How to Reduce Fibromyalgia Symptoms by Reducing Stress

The following are some essential measures you can do to reduce stress and eventually minimize the onset of fibromyalgia symptoms.

Bio-Feedback Therapy

Bio-Feedback therapy is an alternative treatment for fibromyalgia that reduces stress through a special machine which measures the body's response to stress. The purpose of Bio-Feedback is to figure out how your body is reacting to stress, and this knowledge could teach you how to control stress.

Exercise

Whether you participate in a water aerobics class or you are just taking a walk each night before dinner, exercise can improve mental health by curbing anxiety and stress. The classic pain and fatigue caused by fibromyalgia usually prevents many patients from participating in most physical activities that they need to minimize the symptoms. However, exercising - particularly aerobic exercises - can improve a sense of control and could even boost your mood and avoid pain. When you exercise your brain releases endorphins that can act in a similar way to anti-depressants, and this results in a euphoric feeling and lower stress levels.

Relaxation Therapy

This therapy aims to relax the mind and the body through a conscious effort to relax. Even if you do this for only several minutes, you may find this strategy effective at controlling your stress response.

You may want to start by concentrating on one area of your body such as your hands, for example. Focus until you feel that your hands are free of tension or stress. Next, imagine feeling this sensation of weightlessness throughout your body. You can do this while sitting or lying on a comfortable surface. You can dim the lights or shut the lights off and think of a relaxing memory.

Sleep Well

Similar to curbing stress, getting enough sleep at night if you have fibromyalgia is usually more complicated that it appears. This is because fibromyalgia patients usually find it difficult to sleep at night. In addition, high stress and poor sleep can also make the symptoms of fibromyalgia worsen.

Stress and sleep concerns usually come as a pair. If you have sleep problems, you will also likely have high stress levels. But luckily, if you have addressed one, you will also address the other. Getting enough sleep could provide you the chance to experience less stress. And if you experience less stress, you will also find that getting sleep at night will be a lot easier.

There are no strict guidelines when it comes to relaxation. Do anything that will put you in a relaxed mind.

Warm Bath

Warm moisture, either through a warm bath or sitting in a steamy room (sauna) can reduce the release of stress hormones and elevate the levels of endorphins, which serve as natural painkillers. Another benefit of a warm bath is that the heat can relax tensed muscles, so the symptoms of fibromyalgia will be improved.

Find Balance

Finding balance is key in managing stress. In many cases, this refers to having the guts to say no if you think you are being overwhelmed. Find balance in your life and make time for the things that you want to do aside from the things that you must do.

Take note that stress alone doesn't cause fibromyalgia. However, it can definitely make the condition worse. You should take care of yourself and make lifestyle changes so that your fibromyalgia symptoms will be reduced. This will provide you a holistic quality of life.

Chapter 7:
Sleep Strategies for
Fibromyalgia Patients

People who are suffering from fibromyalgia usually experience sleep problems such as insomnia or a difficulty to fall asleep. Some also experience frequent awakenings, which can be remembered the next day. Regular awakenings will disrupt deep sleep. There are also other sleep problems such as sleep apnea and restless legs syndrome that can be linked to fibromyalgia.

Fibromyalgia patients experience waking up every morning feeling tired with low energy. More often than not, they are even more tired during day, and some will go back to sleep during the day to ease their exhaustion. It is also common for fibromyalgia patients to find it difficult to focus during the day, which is known as fibro fog.

Anxiety, depression, pain, and other symptoms of fibromyalgia could also cause sleep problems.

Restless Leg Syndrome and Fibromyalgia

Restless Leg Syndrome is a form of neurologic syndrome distinguished by an overwhelming temptation to move your legs, even at rest. This disorder is very common to people with fibromyalgia. There is an available treatment for this syndrome, so you should consult your doctor if you are suffering from this disorder.

Sleep Strategies to Help Fibromyalgia Patients

Following improved sleep hygiene can help in managing the symptoms of fibromyalgia. Improving your sleep may help in reducing pain, fibro fog and fatigue. You can try the following sleep strategies and check if they can help with your sleep.

- Get the right amount of sleep — no more and no less. Sleep only as much as you need so you can be healthy and refreshed for the following day. Reducing the time in bed could even solidify sleep. Excessive hours in bed may even cause shallow and fragmented sleep.

- Write in a sleep journal. Record how you sleep every night as well as the triggers that could have interrupted your sleep. Reviewing your journal over several weeks could give you overview about your sleep problems.

- Wake up at a regular time every morning. A regular time to rise up can help in fortifying your circadian cycle and will lead to a regular time of sleeping.

- Use relaxation strategies. Deep breathing, gentle massage, and other relaxation strategies can help you in managing fibromyalgia and could help you in improving your sleep.

- Regular exercise can help, but you should avoid exercising three hours before sleep time. In general, exercise can help in improving the quality of your sleep.

- Sound-proof your bedroom, especially if you need silence to achieve enough shut-eye. Loud noises such as loud music or jet flyovers could interfere with sleep even for people who are not experiencing fibromyalgia symptoms.

- Stay away from long naps during the day time. Too much napping could interfere with your night time sleep.

- Lower the temperature in your room. Too much warmth in your room can disturb sleep.

- Hunger can also interfere with sleep. Hence, a light snack at least two hours before sleep time can help in achieving restful sleep.

- Stay away from caffeine or alcohol at night. These will interfere with sleep.

Prescription Drugs for Fibromyalgia

Treatment of fibromyalgia, including its symptoms such as depression and pain can help in easing sleep problems. The prescription drugs approved for fibromyalgia include Savella (milnacipran), Lyrica (pregabalin), and Cymbalta (duloxetine). Other prescription drugs used for fibromyalgia patients in managing symptoms include antidepressants, muscle relaxants, and pain relievers. You can also consult your doctor if you think you may need sleeping pills.

Chapter 8:
Alternative Treatment Options for Fibromyalgia

Limited research has been done on the effectiveness of alternative strategies for fibromyalgia. But many patients with fibromyalgia and some physicians believe that some alternative treatments could help in easing fatigue, pain, and other symptoms, particularly when performed alongside traditional treatment methods.

Dietary Supplements for Fibromyalgia

The following are the available dietary supplements for fibromyalgia:

- S-Adenosyl-L-Methionine (SAMe). This supplement is a derivative of an amino acid, which boosts level of dopamine and serotonin, which are chemicals found in the brain. This supplement can improve sleep and mood.

- 5-Hydroxytrytophan (5-HTP). This supplement is a building block for serotonin. Minimal levels of serotonin are linked to depression. Hence, doctors believe that increasing the levels of serotonin in the body could lead to improved mood. Research has revealed that 5-HTP supplements can also help in easing morning stiffness, fibro pain, insomnia, and anxiety. In the past, supplements containing 5-HTP were linked to a severe disorder known as EMS or eosinophilia-myalgia syndrome. But this is found to be caused by a contaminant in several products.

- Melatonin. This hormone is usually used in nutritional supplements in order to improve sleep. This could also ease pain caused by fibromyalgia.

- Magnesium. Reduced levels of magnesium in the body are associated with fibromyalgia. But based on recent studies, there is no established fact that taking magnesium supplements will help in easing out fibromyalgia symptoms. However, it can also help with sleep so it doesn't hurt to experiment with.

- Saint John's Wort. Even though this herb is often times used to treat specific symptoms of fibromyalgia, there is no established fact that this is effective. Several studies suggest that this might help in easing out mild depression. However, it could also restrict the effectiveness of some prescription drugs used for fibromyalgia. Check this with your Doctor first.

Take note that the idea behind taking alternative dietary supplements is to enhance the levels of specific substances in your body, which might help in fighting fibromyalgia symptoms. Physicians agree that if there is lack of a substance that you can measure, it also makes sense to replace this deficiency.

You should always take extra caution when you are taking supplements for fibromyalgia. You should talk with your doctor, as some supplements could have damaging interactions with your prescription drugs. Some supplements are not safe if you are diagnosed with particular medical disorders. You should always be wary of products that offer relief from fibromyalgia or contain supplements that are not often used in mainstream medication.

Fibromyalgia and Acupuncture

In conventional Chinese medicine, acupuncture is used to rebalance the energy flow in the body. In the West, acupuncture is used to increase the flow of the blood and to improve the production of the natural painkillers of the body.

Acupuncture usually involves stimulating areas of the body by inserting thin needles in the skin. If a small electric current passes through the needles, this is referred to as electro-acupuncture. These methods are both used for fibromyalgia. Some patients find relief from fibromyalgia symptoms through acupuncture. Others have failed to find relief.

Some clinical studies reveal that acupuncture can considerably reduce anxiety and fatigue among fibromyalgia patients. Other studies suggest that acupuncture can ease fibromyalgia pain. However, many studies are conclusive that acupuncture does not ease fibromyalgia symptoms permanently.

Fibromyalgia and Massage Therapy

Massage can ease muscle pain and reduce muscle tension. It can also enhance circulation, improve the production of natural pain relievers in the body, and widen range of motion. Some studies reveal that massage can also boost the patient's mood. It could also help in improving sleep among fibromyalgia patients.

You should take note that there are few studies about the massage effects on fibromyalgia symptoms, and the results are mixed. However, a research study conducted by the Touch Research Institute at the University of Miami reported that even 20 minutes of mild massage could minimize the chemicals linked with stress and pain while also increasing the serotonin production in the body.

Massage can help patients to get a good night's sleep and fight fatigue and fibro fog.

Home Treatments for Fibromyalgia

There are also simple and affordable home treatments for fibromyalgia pain. Remember, heat — particularly moisture heat — could temporarily ease stiffness and pain by increasing blood flow to the body areas where you are feeling pain.

You can apply a warm moist pad, warm your clothes in the dryer, or take a hot bath. Using cold pads can also help you feel better by minimizing the muscle pain caused by fibromyalgia.

Chapter 9:
Changing Your Perception
About Fibromyalgia

Viewing fibromyalgia from a different angle like referring to it as something that you have, instead of something that you are, could help you assess your life and consider about what you could do in opposition to what you can't do.

Even though undergoing medically recommended therapies and alternative medicines may not completely cure the symptoms of fibromyalgia for you, they can be used to minimize the symptoms, which is often helpful in getting your life back on track. There is no miracle cure for fibromyalgia, but with the ability to control and reduce the symptoms, while still living your life is a great way to ensure that you come out as the victor against fibromyalgia.

The Role of Optimism Against Fibromyalgia

Optimism is essential if you want to regain control of your life, and your condition. The way that you perceive your condition, and the way that you allow it to affect your life can have a significant impact on your overall well-being.

Viewing your fibromyalgia from a different angle, embracing it for what it is, then learning how to cope with it, can make your life more satisfying. One way to beat down fibromyalgia is through reframing.

Reframing refers to a psychological strategy, which entails looking at something from a new angle. Viewing fibromyalgia from a new perspective can provide you more optimism, for instance, if your neck is aching, instead of focusing on how painful it is, you should find new avenues to think differently.

Instead of thinking that you are in so much pain, and you don't know when or even if you will ever experience relief from all the pain, you can instead tell yourself that if you do some stretches, have a warm bath, and rest, that you will find relief.

Viewing your pain, your condition, and your other symptoms from a better view, can help you see the lighter side of things and deal with your present condition much more effectively.

Living a Happy Life Even with Fibromyalgia

One of the best ways for you to feel better about your life even with fibromyalgia is to think about what you do have. Aim to focus on your blessings, and how these blessings can transform your life for the better.

People with fibromyalgia find it easy to feel sorry for their situation, especially if the pain and lethargy are unbearable. However, thinking about what you could do, instead of what you cannot do, is a great way to avoid negative thinking.

Another way for you to build a more satisfying life is for you to pursue new hobbies. Doing activities that help you to focus on something other than your fibromyalgia pain can greatly help you.

Taking Care of Yourself First

Many people with fibromyalgia forget to take care of themselves. This is often the case for patients with families to take care for, and work obligations that may eat up a lot of their time.

Those who are suffering from fibromyalgia should take care of themselves first, even if they are already accustomed of the pain and the tiredness of every day life. Looking after yourself includes getting enough rest and getting the support you need from your family and friends.

Learning how you can look after yourself and understanding that doing so could help you feel better is the primary step in achieving relief from all of the symptoms.

Know Your Limits

Knowing your limits is vital if you want to regain control of your life. You should understand that you may not be able to do as much as you like, but you should also understand that this is totally okay!

Below are some pointers you can follow to help you establish limits and regain control of your life:

It's Okay to Say No

If you are regularly asked to visit a place to do something, you should not feel obliged to be there always if you really can't make it. Take note that you have a serious physical condition, and you should prioritize it. Don't be depressed if you can't go to see your friends, or partake in a particular activity because of your symptoms. Simply focus on improving and getting better each day until you reach a point where you no longer have to say no.

Write in a Journal

A good way to understand what is setting your fibromyalgia off is to write about it in a journal. You can record the number of hours you have slept during the previous night, what type of food you have eaten, what medications you have taken, and activities that you have performed. A closer look at what you have been doing recently could help you to determine problems and will encourage you to stay away from things that could stress you out.

Ask For Assistance

It's perfectly fine to ask for help. This doesn't signify that you are a weak person, and it's not a sign that you can't be well. Your family and friends are always there to help you. You just need to let them know what you need to do, what you need, and how they can help you. Soon, you will find that they will also be more understanding if your situation is really bad.

Assign House Chores

Because women are more prone to acquiring fibromyalgia, many find it hard to deal with it especially if they need to do house chores. Hence, you should delegate the tasks to your housemates. Let your family members know and understand your situation, so they can help out with chores, especially if you are in pain. If your family is aware that you find it hard to do the house chores, they will be more understanding and more than willing to help.

Take Enough Rest

There are times that you need to step aside and rest. It is even recommended to take a bit of time out from your usual activities for several days on occasion. A few days of deep rest will do you wonders.

Be Active Whenever You Can

When you need to get out and do a bit of strenuous activity, be sure that you only do so if you're feeling up to it. That is why keeping a journal is crucial as you will know the best hours that your body is fit for any activity. Exercise when you are well, and you can follow a schedule around your peak hours. Doing this will help you to do more things as well as help you feel better about yourself.

Conclusion

Thanks again for taking the time to read this book!

You should now have a good understanding of fibromyalgia, and have some strategies for treating and improving it.

I wish you the best of luck in your battle against fibromyalgia. Remember to stay positive, and that you're not alone. Many others are fighting the same battle that you are, and many have managed to overcome it! Keep on fighting, have the right mental attitude, and you too will be able to achieve relief from fibromyalgia!

If you enjoyed this book, please take the time to leave me a review on Amazon. I appreciate your honest feedback, and it really helps me to continue producing high quality books.